REVERSE DIABETES: THE NATURAL WAY

How To Be Diabetes-Free In 21 Days
7 Step Success System

RANDALL VINCENT-MARTIN

ISBN: 1536890855
ISBN-13: 978-1536890853

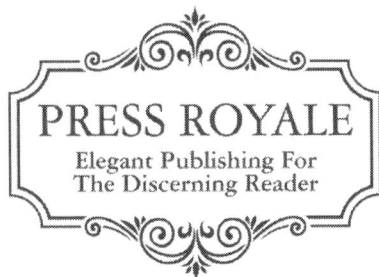

PRESS ROYALE

Elegant Publishing For
The Discerning Reader

WELCOME TO
"REVERSE DIABETES: THE NATURAL WAY"

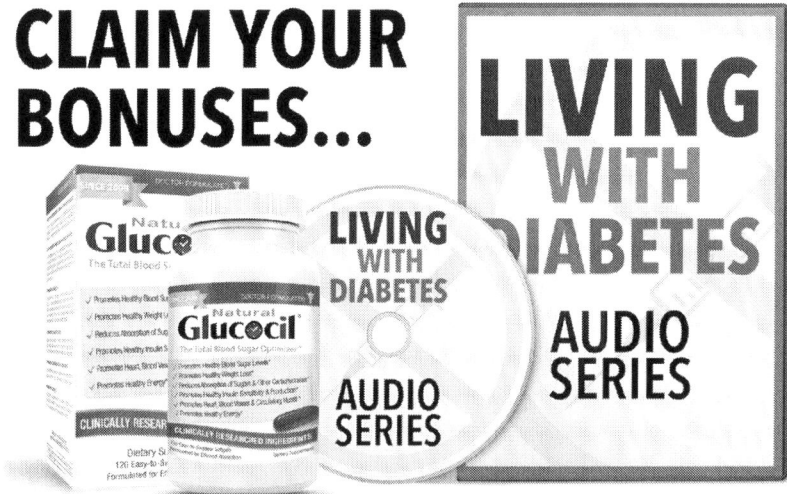

Every copy of this book comes packed with these valuable bonuses:

BONUS #1
Glucocil Natural Blood Sugar Optimizer - **15 DAY SAMPLE**

BONUS #2
"Living With Diabetes" Audio Series - **FREE INSTANT DOWNLOAD**

BONUS #3
"Diabetes & You" Weekly Newsletter - **FREE INSTANT ACCESS**

Simply visit the special URL below and enter your name & email address for instant access.

pressroyale.com/claim

RANDALL VINCENT-MARTIN

CONTENTS

INTRODUCTION

Welcome to the essential guide to reversing type-2 diabetes the natural way.

In this book, you will learn about the signs, symptoms, causes, and drug-free preventatives, as well as reversal methods you can use in order to improve your life or a loved one's.

Educating yourself is the first step. Putting what you learn into practice is the next and last.

It's that simple.

Remember the three main areas of promoting positive well-being: healthy diet, physical activity, and stress reduction.

When you implement these three categories together there is no room left for diabetes.

That is the bare bones fact of permanently reversing diabetes.

In order to faithfully make this transition and stick to it permanently, it is necessary to be honest with yourself where you are currently at with your eating habits, indulgent tendencies, physical activity or inactivity and stress triggers.

You will only be cheating yourself if you try to rationalize out of any one of these areas.

Keep a chart or poster of your goals where you can see it and read it every day.

Make it a habit of putting everything else on hold and taking a few moments for yourself to review the goals that you really want and to be proud of yourself for taking the necessary steps.

Repetition truly does help plant the seeds of positive change.

It is a mental game as much or even more so as it is a physical game of transforming your habits.

Try to be easy on yourself by implementing the changes gradually rather than taking it on all at once.

Finding the pace that works for you, even if it is slow, is going to be the most effective and helpful thing that you can do for yourself.

Seek out support systems that encourage you to keep steadily along your path, whether they are family and friends, social groups, or programs dedicated to seeing you become a confident success in reaching your goals.

You *can* do this and now that you have educated yourself with the essential knowledge to transform your life into one you *want*, all you have to do is walk through the door to action; actualize it, one step at a time.

Read it cover to cover.

Take action.

And this book really can change your life.

To your success,

Randall Vincent-Martin

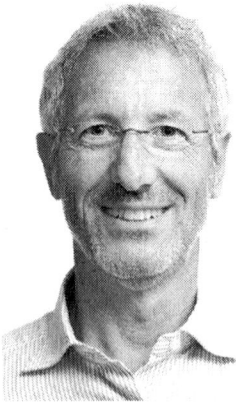

IS IT REALLY POSSIBLE TO REVERSE DIABETES NATURALLY?

Doug, from Salt Lake City, Utah said:

*"I felt **overwhelmed** by my diabetes. I was always tired at work, and I couldn't keep up with my kids anymore! Just the thought of vacation, or even a day on the town, made me feel exhausted. Diabetes made me feel **like a prisoner in my own life**.*

I'm so glad I found this <u>scientifically proven</u> way to reverse my Type-2 diabetes. It's <u>not</u> untested, junk science. It's a proven, practical method to jumpstart your pancreas and get your body to regulate your blood sugar again.

I'm living proof that it works... I haven't needed diabetes medication for over 6 months!

*Everybody with Type 2 diabetes needs to watch this video **right now**, so they can reverse their diabetes in just a few weeks."*

Andrew from Battleground, Washington wrote:

*"... showed me the **simple solution** to my diabetes, and you had **the science to back it up**.*

I thought I'd be stuck with Type-2 diabetes forever. But now I've been diabetes-free almost 18 months.

My doctor was shocked when I told him that I hadn't needed an insulin shot for weeks. He had to test my blood sugar himself to believe it.

The best part is, I used what I discovered… to **jumpstart my pancreas** *and reverse my diabetes in just 17 days!"*

They are just two regular guys that reversed their type-2 diabetes naturally.

Read on to find out more… and don't miss the **Shortcut System in the final chapter of this book.**

WHAT IS DIABETES?

Type-2 diabetes, just like type-1 diabetes, is not a direct disease inflicted upon the body but rather a group of related disorders that are identified primarily by disruptions in the body's ability to metabolize glucose.

Glucose is a broken-down form of sugars that the body is designed to absorb for cells' use as energy reserves to keep us going throughout the day.

These sugars commonly come from the foods and drinks that we consume, but when absolutely necessary the body can metabolize them from fats stored in the body as well as muscle fibers.

In a person with diabetes, there can be a number of different disturbances going on with this metabolic process.

The issue could be the pancreas's reduced ability to produce insulin, a hormone that helps the body's cells absorb glucose from the bloodstream.

Or it could be an issue with the cells' ability to actually uptake glucose, even though the pancreas is producing enough insulin. Or it could be a combination of the two.

The difference between type-1 and type-2 diabetes is that type-1 is an autoimmune disease, meaning it has hereditary implications and the immune system cells of the afflicted person actually attack their own pancreas where insulin is produced.

The elimination of these insulin-producing cells causes a lifelong deficiency of insulin, as far as doctors currently know, and requires people with type-1 to become dependent on insulin supplements.

Type-2 diabetes is not autoimmune related. It is seen as a reversible condition that is usually turned around by a few small but crucial lifestyle changes in diet and exercise.

The exact cause that leads to type-2 is not known, but it is obvious that for some, a diet high in carbs and excessive sugars wears out the pancreas over time.

In others, an inactive lifestyle contributes to a sluggish metabolism and high blood sugar levels.

Some cases show that while insulin levels are normal, a high influx of glucose is too much for the body to process while other cases reveal that target cells in the body meant to uptake glucose are lacking the necessary receptor sites to receive insulin.

The complications that arise from diabetes are vast and depend in seriousness on how far along the condition has persisted before diagnosis.

Frequent urination, excessive thirst, hunger and atherosclerosis (plaque buildup in the arterial walls as well as other blood vessels) are the most common results.

If gone unchecked or untreated, this disease can lead to cardiovascular disease, kidney disease, impaired vision, nerve damage, ulcers, edema, and even amputation.

Diabetes is actually the reason for roughly 82,000 lower extremity amputations per year in the US alone.

Conventional treatments for type-2 diabetes, as already mentioned, are dietary changes like the reduction of carb intake and reduction or elimination of sugar additives, and sugary foods and drinks.

Exercise regimens also promote reversal by keeping the body active and burning up those excess sugars in the circulatory system.

Patients are encouraged to transition at their own pace, but diligently, so there are really no cons to these approaches.

In addition, many patients are asked to keep their blood sugars under control with a blood-checking monitor and supplemental insulin doses.

While these definitely aid in supervising and controlling blood sugar levels, test strips, lancets, and supplements could be considered too costly to become a regular expense.

Prevention and maintenance toward reversal are the best options and can be administered through self-care and natural solutions.

Even so, the road to recovery can surely be challenging at times and therefore is greatly alleviated by organized support programs that provide further education and step-by-step action.

You can find our list of recommended support programs at the back of the book.

THE 7 RISK FACTORS FOR TYPE-2 DIABETES

The following are the seven most common risk factors that contribute to diabetes type-2.

Observe and avoid these and you will already be well on your way to reversing and abstaining from the onset of this disease.

Every action that you take toward recognizing these risk factors will add to the momentum and sustainability of your regulated blood sugars as well as your overall health.

Risk #1: Weight

This is a huge contributor as about 90% of people at the time of diagnosis are obese. Obesity means that a person's weight is at least 20% higher than it should be according to the body mass index chart.

It basically reveals the sufferer of the condition that one's body weight is comprised of an excessive percentage of fat, enough to cause health risks in a number of different areas, including diabetes type-2.

The body mass index (BMI) figures depend on one's age, weight and height. Online BMI calculators that will help you determine your ideal weight and what your current BMI figure is.

According to the BMI chart, being overweight begins at a figure of 25 while obesity starts at 30. (There is a free online BMI calculator in the Links section at the back of the book).

Risk #2: High Blood Glucose

Blood glucose levels relay just how much sugar is floating around in the blood without being picked up and absorbed by the body's cells.

Every time we consume food and drinks our blood sugar levels rise a bit until the body has had time to absorb glucose from the bloodstream into the cells for energy conversion.

Whenever we become active by simply moving about for at least 20 minutes or engaging in exercise, our blood sugar levels begin to drop because that glucose is being converted into energy to keep us going.

Foods high in starch, simple carbohydrates and sugar as well as natural juices contribute to blood sugar spikes that provide energy for a short time (one to two hours) but get burned up so quickly in the metabolic process of healthy people that it leaves us experiencing a sugar crash.

On the other hand, complex carbohydrates metabolize more slowly in the body providing a more sustainable source of energy.

There are a couple ways to measure blood glucose levels.

One is a fasting blood sugar check, which means testing with a conventional blood checker at least four hours after consuming anything other than water.

You can find over the counter fasting blood sugar devices online or at any drug store (See the Shopping List section at the back of the book).

The most accurate test is done in a lab where blood is drawn after a person that has fasted for at least eight hours, and it is called an A1C test.

A normal reading for the quick blood testing device is anywhere from 80 to 110, while a normal reading for the A1C test is between 4% and 5.9%.

When A1C tests show 6% or more, doctors diagnose the patient as having diabetes.

Risk #3: High Blood Pressure

This is a simple concept that most all of us are already aware of.

Stress, dehydration, excessive sodium in the diet, and excessive consumption of foods high in fat and cholesterol all contribute to high blood pressure.

The heart is working harder than usual to make sure that blood is getting pumped to every area of the body, making sure that the cells stay nourished, oxygenated, and healthy.

You can easily check your blood pressure by purchasing an inexpensive monitor online or at any drug store, (see the Shopping List section at the back of the book) but they usually have one available near the pharmacy allowing you to check it on the spot.

Normal levels for a person at rest are 120/80. Any strenuous activity, including exercise and simple emotional stress, contribute to high blood pressure.

The longer that a person remains in a stressful or traumatic state, whether they are aware of it or not, the higher the risk factor they have for developing constant high blood pressure conditions.

Remember not to sweat the small stuff and keep calm!

Risk #4: Unhealthy Cholesterol

There are two types of cholesterol: HDLs (High-Density Lipoproteins (or fats) and LDLs (Low-Density Lipoproteins).

Each of these occurs naturally in the bloodstream but they must be balanced in order to stay healthy.

HDLs are the good kind that regulates LDL storage and enforces excretion by helping to remove excess LDLs from blood vessel walls.

LDLs are the unwanted kind that stores cholesterol in the blood stream, causing plaque buildup.

The cholesterol buildup taxes smooth blood flow, putting a strain on the heart which can lead to a number of further complications, including high blood pressure, cardiovascular disease, aneurysm, embolism, blood clotting, heart attack, and stroke, among others.

Again, both types of cholesterol can be easily checked at home using an inexpensive kit – see the Shopping List section at the back of the book.

Risk #5: Physical Inactivity

This contributor involves any type of lifestyle that gets the heart rate up through physical activity for at least 20 to 30 minutes per day.

By working jobs that have us sitting in a chair for a good part of the day, sitting in cars and then coming home to rest and perhaps sit in front of the TV for entertainment before going to bed and doing it all over again the next day, we are required to be more mindful about engaging the body.

Without doing so, a habit of physical inactivity leads to sluggish and stagnating organ function.

Over a long enough period of time, it can also foster the deterioration of certain organs and body structures caused by lack of stimulation.

This is why it becomes a concern and a determining factor in causing type-2 diabetes.

Risk #6: Smoking

Perhaps it goes without saying that there is absolutely nothing healthy about smoking.

Even for those who are trying to "smoke healthy" by buying additive-free tobacco brands, they are as equally affected by the negative repercussions.

Smoking contributes to atherosclerosis (plaque buildup in the arteries and veins) from cholesterol as well as tar.

It reduces organ function because of excessive carbon monoxide and carbon dioxide levels in the bloodstream and body, depleting oxygen levels.

Furthermore, smoking causes poor circulation throughout the body, lessening and eventually cutting off blood flow to the extremities.

This is a dangerous combination for patients who have diabetes because they are already prone to edema, gout, and reduced circulation to the legs and feet.

Risk #7: Unhealthy Eating

As a brief overview, foods that are high in carbs, enriched flour, sugar, sodium, fats and grease, unhealthy oils, as well as processed foods are all considered unhealthy when they become a staple in anyone's diet.

These are all foods that should be consumed sparingly. Even seemingly healthy foods like potatoes, white rice, pasta, and whole grain bread still possess those simple carbs that only convert to quickly processed sugars in the body, providing little actual nutrition while promoting high blood glucose levels.

It's not always about what one eats, but also how much one eats.

This especially goes along with a person's activity levels in their daily routine.

If a person is living a relatively sedentary lifestyle while consuming more than three meals and two snacks per day or are eating more than four to five ounces of meat and over one cup of carb source per meal, they are overdoing it.

While each individual requires a relatively different diet.

Depending on your body type, moderation is the key that you can use in your life as a diabetic.

STEP 1:
HOW TO LOSE WEIGHT WITHOUT REALLY NOTICING

No matter your tactical approach to losing weight, consistency is the underlying theme that leads to success.

You do not need a gym membership, nor do you need to push yourself to the limits to shed pounds. In fact, healthy weight loss is only the loss of one to two pounds lost per week.

Weight loss can truly begin with something as easy as changing your diet.

Cut out fast food and processed foods bought from the grocery store.

Centralize your diet around eating plenty of vegetables as well as high-protein and low-fat meats like poultry and fish.

Salmon, mackerel, halibut, cod, and tuna, as well as sardines, are great examples.

Invest in raw nuts like pecans, walnuts, and almonds. Likewise, you can eat seeds such as pumpkin, sunflower, and sesame seeds for snacking.

Small amounts of dried fruits will add flavor to your snacking experience, but be wary as there are many varieties preserved in excessive amounts of sugar.

The elimination of soft drinks can create huge results!

Instead of going out to eat frequently, look up easy-to-make recipes online or invest in a healthy cookbook or two, and prepare meals over the weekend that will last you throughout the week.

This will not only help you lose weight, it will cut down on preparation time during your weekdays and can save you a noticeable amount of money.

Aside from dietary changes, make it a point to engage in some kind of physical activity every single day.

Start out easy on yourself to keep up your confidence and motivation, helping to change your perspective about exercise by realizing that it doesn't have to be strenuous and can actually be enjoyable.

Taking walks for at least 20 minutes per day, swimming, cycling, and even doing household chores that keep you up and active, are all ways that contribute to successive weight loss without really noticing that you are putting out a lot of effort.

It is amazing how many calories can be burned through vacuuming, mowing the lawn, and making beds.

While you are encouraged to set your own pace and empower yourself with your own decision-making process, it helps to join programs that support your motives.

There are organizations out there that have had years of experience and knowledge in order to help people consolidate their efforts for weight loss and diabetes reversal to a streamlined process.

Remember that you are not alone in self-improvement and participating with other people in a similar position makes the process that much more fun!

You can find a list of recommended support programs at the back of the book.

SUMMARY & ACTION PLAN

1. Cut out processed and fast foods

2. Prepare healthy food at home with healthy ingredients

3. Take 20 minutes exercise a day

4. Look at joining recommended support programs (see list at back of book).

STEP 2:
HOW TO LOWER YOUR BLOOD GLUCOSE LEVEL AND STILL EAT DESSERTS

Once you have a consistent exercise routine in place that keeps you active and your body systems stimulated, you have set the foundation for keeping your blood glucose levels in check.

Physical activity draws upon energy sources within the body, namely glucose, and automatically coerces the body into drawing up those glucose levels from the body to help reduce high blood sugars.

The American Diabetes Association (ADA) recommend these ten superfoods:

1. Beans
2. Dark green leafy vegetables
3. Citrus fruit
4. Sweet potatoes
5. Berries
6. Tomatoes
7. Fish high in Omega-3 fatty acids
8. Whole grains
9. Nuts
10. Fat-free milk and yoghurt

The ADA also recommends avoiding sugary drinks like regular soda, fruit punch, fruit drinks, energy drinks, and sweet tea, as they will raise your blood glucose levels and can provide several hundred calories in just a single serving.

A 12-ounce can of regular soda has about 150 calories and 40 grams of carbohydrate.

This is the same amount of carbohydrate in a staggering 10 teaspoons of sugar.

They instead suggest zero-calorie or very low-calorie drinks, including

- Water
- Unsweetened teas
- Coffee (preferably decaffeinated)
- Diet soda
- Other low-calorie drinks and drink mixes

There is a medical field called Naturopathy that believes in healing patients through nutrition.

Patients who have faithfully stuck to the regimens provided by these practicing doctors, known as Naturopaths, have seen complete reversals and recoveries from all sorts of diseases, including type-2 diabetes.

Some of the recommendations provided by such doctors in the growing field of Naturopathy incorporate particular spices and herbs that can either be taken as supplements or added into cooked meals.

These spices, herbs and other food sources that have once been overlooked are now being highly regarded for their positive and health-promoting effects on the body.

Cinnamon, for example, is great for helping to reduce high blood pressure and blood sugar levels.

Fresh garlic does the same, along with containing antioxidant properties that remove free radicals from the body.

Turmeric and fresh ginger are anti-inflammatories that help to greatly improve and regulate digestive health; the digestive system is seen as being a regulator for overall bodily health.

It makes sense since it's through the digestive system that we absorb all of our nutrients to sustain vitality, while, in turn, inflammation within the body is rapidly being recognized as a major contributor and source to a widespread number of diseases.

By greatly reducing and moderating high-carb and sugary foods and drinks, you establish a healthy, supportive diet that leaves room for a little indulgence here and there.

Desserts should still be taken in moderation, and they do not even have to be the overzealous sugar bombs that we are used to consuming like cheesecake or candy bars.

Believe it or not, there are actually 'healthy' desserts out there that you can even make yourself in no time at all.

See the Links section at the back of the book for some of our favorite diabetic desserts.

And lastly, a simple way to help regulate your blood glucose level is by taking natural supplements, such as Glucocil.

If you haven't done this already, you can claim a 15-day trial via the link at the front of this book.

SUMMARY & ACTION PLAN

1. Regularly check your blood glucose level / invest in a blood glucose checker*

2. Incorporate superfoods and recommended herbs & spices into your meals

3. Avoid sugary drinks and high-carb foods

4. Take recommended dosage of Glucocil

*See Shopping List at the back of this book

STEP 3:
HOW TO LOWER YOUR BLOOD PRESSURE WITHOUT MEDS

There are a number of different tactics that can be implemented to help keep your blood pressure in check that don't involve drugs.

Sometimes foods are the best medicinal cure, and often they are the best preventative.

Along with eating foods made from cinnamon, turmeric, garlic, and ginger, start incorporating fresh lemon wedges in your drinking water.

Water sustains life, and yet we are all prone to taking it for granted because of how flavorless it is.

Did you know that high blood pressure, high blood glucose, as well as a number of other illnesses like chronic fatigue, irritability, muscle soreness, and sleeplessness, can all be due to something as simple as dehydration?

Make sure that you are getting at least the standard eight glasses of water per day.

Know that stimulants like coffee, sports drinks, energy drinks, sugar in any form, as well as smoking, all cause dehydration (and contribute to high blood pressure).

It's been said that for every cup of coffee you drink, you must drink two glasses of water to balance the effects of the dehydration it causes.

Very important – one of the greatest factors that contribute to high blood pressure is *stress*.

Identify the triggers that make you stressful and avoid them if at all possible.

Engage in programs that promote maintaining calm states of mind.

Everybody is different so it may take some trial and error to find the best method that works for you.

Some examples are yoga, meditation, and massage.

It will be plenty worth the effort because *you* are worth it and so is your health.

Once you have found a method that works it will keep giving back to you for the rest of your life.

Consider also that if you are not able to be in a healthy state, it will be harder for you to be there for your loved ones, so it's important to take care of yourself first.

Experiment with various breath work modalities that provide exercises for regulated breathing, recommend by Deepak Chopra MD and Christiane Northrup MD.

When we get stressed, we stop breathing regularly.

This gives way to stress on our cells and internal organs, especially the heart and brain function.

It causes abnormalities in our sleep patterns that can contribute to difficulty sleeping, insomnia, and sleep apnea, all of which can lead to high blood pressure.

SUMMARY & ACTION PLAN

1. Regularly check your blood pressure / invest in a blood pressure monitor*

2. Drink eight glasses of water a day

3. Eat foods containing cinnamon, turmeric, garlic or ginger

4. Lower stress with yoga, meditation, massage or breath work

*See Shopping List at the back of this book

STEP 4:
HOW TO AVOID UNHEALTHY CHOLESTEROL AND STILL ENJOY FOOD

Juicy burgers, buttery popcorn, and sugary donuts are undeniably delicious, acting like a warm blanket to coat and saturate the taste buds on a cold night.

They have an addictive quality indeed, however the compromise for sating that taste and comfort is havoc wreaked on the lining of the gut, the heart, and arteries, as well as a number of other organs.

Not only that, without our realizing it, we are contributing to a self-defeating principle of feeding an addiction of 'comfort foods' that actually cause us more anxiety, mood swings, fatigue, cloudy thinking and ill-health that adds to the stress in our lives.

Food does not have to layer us with a heavy, saturated blanket of cholesterol in order to enjoy it for all it's worth.

Equally divine tasting oils that provide healthy fats like omega-3's, as well as anti-bacterial and antiseptic properties, are coconut, sesame, avocado, and olive oil.

Cook with these instead, and make sure the label reads "first cold pressed" to ensure that you are getting all of the quality attributes out of them.

Dress up your salads with them; cook your eggs and meats with them; replace vegetable or canola oils with them in recipes and you will be doing your body (and your taste buds) the world of good.

Unhealthy cholesterol comes from red meats like beef, pork and, lamb, fried foods, hydrogenated or partially hydrogenated oils like vegetable, canola, palm, and kernel oils, as well as many processed foods.

Read the nutrition labels on food packages to know how much cholesterol per serving you are getting.

If you are a fan of red meats, feel free to eat them once in a while. When shopping for red meat, look for a ratio of 90% lean to 10% fat.

That way you'll be able to enjoy their taste without soaking up loads of the cholesterol aftermath.

Remember also that there are 1,000 ways to cook chicken and over 1,000 fish in the sea that are great for eating, so you're bound to find a few that speak to your palate.

Do not underestimate the power and sensuous persuasion of adding spices to your meals.

You will always be able to conjure up a plethora of flavors to help make bland foods exciting.

Beyond the conventional salt and pepper shakers, you can throw a dash of paprika on your eggs or salmon; rosemary, thyme, and oregano can complement your chicken; turmeric, cumin and, coriander can spice up a veggie stir-fry.

The possibilities are endless and the benefits are befitting – remember the healthful effects of these food additions will work for your body in ridding it of illness.

SUMMARY & ACTION PLAN

1. Regularly check your cholesterol / invest in a home cholesterol kit*

2. Avoid food containing unhealthy cholesterol

3. Consume more Omega-3 oils

*See Shopping List at the back of this book

STEP 5:
HOW TO GET PHYSICALLY ACTIVE WITHOUT A GYM MEMBERSHIP

We need to promote physical exertion in our daily routine to stimulate the muscles and organs, including the brain.

Indeed, the brain and our mental approach are really where it all starts.

Sometimes even just adjusting our perspective on exercise and what we consider it to entail will turn the typically dreaded feeling that most have about it into something to look forward to.

A recent study by Harvard psychologist Ellen Langer was conducted on hotel maids and the routine chores of their job to see just how much our perspectives determine control over the state of our bodies.

Essentially one group of maids was informed about how many calories were burned for every chore they engaged in while another group was simply left to do their work.

All participants were asked about their physical activity at home, which was relatively minimal.

All maids were asked not to change any of their activity or eating habits for a number of months while this study was being conducted.

At the conclusion of the study, those maids who were informed of the calorie-burning effects of their chores saw a loss of five pounds or more, while the uninformed group saw no change.

The key to getting active and staying that way on a consistent basis is to accept your current weight and health.

If you let your ambitions carry you further than you're currently capable of, you're bound to lose motivation quickly because you've set the standard too high and will end up resenting trying to live up to it every time you exercise.

Start with what you know, and more importantly, start with what you *enjoy*.

That's why going for a walk is highly recommended for people who are not used to being active.

The outdoors is stimulating, you are breathing fresh air, and you're free to go at your own pace.

During the cold months, you can do your walking in a building like a museum, library, department store, and so on.

Again, look to programs that already have participants involved where you can get support and companionship in your efforts.

You can be sure to find local groups in your area and can get involved in all kinds of activities, such as bicycling tours through your town, recreational sports, dance lessons, tame versions of yoga for beginners or anything that entices you to get out of your house and move around.

It is guaranteed that you will find an inviting group out there that is doing something you've always wanted to but didn't know how or is doing something you enjoy and didn't have the support to make it happen.

SUMMARY & ACTION PLAN

1. Take 20 minutes exercise a day

2. Join a Walking Group in your area (see Support Groups section at back of book)

3. Find your favorite venue for exercise to stay motivated

STEP 6:
HOW TO GIVE UP SMOKING WITHOUT PATCHES, GUM OR SPRAY

This is by far the most addictive habit to break, seeing as cigarette smoking has been compared to having similar addictive qualities to cocaine and heroin.

That especially goes for all the additives that are put into tobacco to biologically encourage smokers to keep up the habit.

Fret not because it has been done countless times!

Smoking with vaporizers or e-cigarettes is the most modern method of helping smokers quit as they eliminate the highly addictive additives that are put into tobacco cigarettes.

They consist mainly of nicotine and with the cartridges that are offered on the market, several varying degrees of nicotine percentages are offered to help wean off of the habit.

This method is a gradual, stepped-down program like the patches or gum that still provide smokers with the oral fixation of smoking without the off-putting smell, although it is still costly and it still introduces addictive nicotine into the body.

Nicotine affects the nervous system of the body and stimulates serotonin production in the brain.

Serotonin is that 'feel good' hormone that is really what keeps smokers going back for more.

The usual stories relate smokers to taking up the habit whenever they are stressed out and need a break or oftentimes when they are confronted with a certain 'wait period', whether it is driving in the car, transitioning from one activity to the next or some other lull in their daily routine.

One effective way to quit smoking is to mimic the same procedure that patches or gum offer by stepping down the number of cigarettes you consume per day.

Start with your usual amount then gradually reduce that amount by one to two cigarettes each day per week.

You can allot yourself a certain amount and leave the rest at home and remain faithful to only smoking that allotted amount.

Carry toothpicks with you and pop one in your mouth every time you feel the need for a cigarette.

To get the same serotonin boost that nicotine provides, engage in physical activity each day instead.

This will help to reverse the circulatory damage that smoking causes, as well as provide you with the same 'feel good' hormonal boost that the nicotine gives.

Physical exercise has been proven to be a serotonin producer, so it will be killing two birds with one stone so-to-speak in dropping a bad habit and replacing it with a good one, as well as keeping your blood sugar levels in check.

A problem most people have with giving up smoking is missing the physical action of holding and putting a cigarette in your mouth.

Getting rid of the psychological addiction can be as hard as the physical addiction.

This problem can be resolved with a nicotine-free dummy or harmless from companies such as InfuseAir.

Oftentimes, the cravings seem so strong that smokers tend to give into them.

Remember, the cravings will pass.

Stay focused on what you truly want for yourself during these times and, day by day, your resolve to abstain will become stronger.

SUMMARY & ACTION PLAN

1. Gradually reduce the amount you smoke daily

2. Invest in a nicotine-free smoking substitute*

3. Replace missing serotonin with exercise

4. Join a stop smoking support group (see Support Groups section at back of book)

*See Shopping List at the back of this book

STEP 7:
HOW TO EAT HEALTHILY AND STILL ENJOY EVERY MEAL & SNACK

Enjoying a life of healthy eating at every meal and snack is not a difficult task; it simply requires a few small changes to your routine.

This is going to require you to up your cooking game a bit.

Once you get into it, you will be glad that you did - and will soon realize just how fulfilling healthy food can be.

Filling your body with the right foods will leave you feeling energized to get everything done in your day that you've set out to do rather than eating unhealthy foods that compromise your energy and leave you reaching for coffee, energy drinks, or sugary snacks just to keep going for a couple hours and crash again later.

Most importantly, within the first couple weeks of dedicating yourself to a healthy diet regimen, you will notice an elevation in your mood and clearer thinking.

A healthy body means a healthy mind.

In order to continue to give your taste buds that sweet comfort, you can supplement your meals and snacks with natural sweeteners that have a much lower glycemic index (sugar content per gram) than refined white sugars.

Refined sugars, by the way, are literal poison to the body, just as high fructose corn syrups, and they should be avoided at all costs.

Mercury has been found in almost a third of the 55 most popular food and beverage products that have high fructose corn syrup as their first or second highest ingredient, according to a Princeton research team.

You will not be missing out by removing them from your diet!

Instead, incorporate a little organic honey or pure maple syrup on your toasted oats in the morning or use them to replace sugar when called for in recipes.

Agave sweetener and stevia, a plant that is naturally 400 times sweeter than sugar, are other healthier choices to accent your food.

There is an awe-inspiring world of easy-to-make recipes that the masses at large are not privy to yet because we are so conditioned to a fast-paced lifestyle that leaves us buying whatever pre-packaged, ready-made, processed foods are available in the grocery aisle.

We are giving up our health and well-being for tasteful satisfaction and time savers, but it doesn't have to be so.

Invest in a healthy cookbook or make your own from your healthily-converted recipes sought online.

Look for supportive dietary programs that cater to your diabetes-reversing needs and always, don't forget to read the nutrition labels and ingredients lists to get a good idea of what exactly you are putting into your body.

One great rule of thumb to go by when preparing meals is "the fresher, the better".

You usually can't do better than organic meats and vegetables.

SUMMARY & ACTION PLAN

1. Replace refined sugars with natural sweeteners*

2. Avoid all food or drinks that contains high-fructose corn syrup

3. Read a healthy recipe book, and try something new

4. Join a diabetes support group (see Support Groups section at back of book)

*See Shopping List at the back of this book

WHAT WILL YOUR FUTURE HOLD? THE FOUR OPTIONS

We've done our part in sharing this information with you, so now it's your turn to make a decision.

As you can now see, it really is possible to reverse diabetes naturally.

You now have four possible options to choose from:

Option 1: WORST OUTCOME

You can ignore the advice you have read in this book; ignore the advice you have been given by your doctor or medical professional, and carry on eating and drinking the same diet and lifestyle – and suffer the potentially deadly outcome.

Option 2: REASONABLE OUTCOME

You can follow the advice of your medical professional and do everything he/she tells you, and spend the rest of your life managing your diabetes with expensive medication, but never actually recovering from the disease.

Option 3: BEST OUTCOME

You can follow the advice of your medical professional and do everything he/she tells you, **AND** follow all 7 of the steps outlined in this book, and you will be on the sure path to reversing your diabetes.

Option 4: ULTIMATE SOLUTION

Follow the advice of your medical professional and do everything he/she tells you, while at the same time following all 7 of the steps outlined in this book.

That's really all you need to do.

But many of us already struggle to manage our current daily routines of chores, family, work and errands.

So if this sounds like you, there is **a MASSIVE, time-saving, life-extending shortcut**.

Read the next section to find out more…

THE SHORTCUT TO PERMANENTLY REVERSING DIABETES IN 3 WEEKS

At the start of this book, we shared these testimonials with you:

*"I felt **overwhelmed** by my diabetes. I was always tired at work, and I couldn't keep up with my kids anymore! Just the thought of vacation, or even a day on the town, made me feel exhausted. Diabetes made me feel **like a prisoner in my own life**.*

I'm so glad I found this scientifically proven way to reverse my Type 2 diabetes. It's not untested, junk science. It's a proven, practical method to jumpstart your pancreas and get your body to regulate your blood sugar again.

I'm living proof that it works… I haven't needed diabetes medication for over 6 months!

*Everybody with Type 2 diabetes needs to watch this video **right now**, so they can reverse their diabetes in just a few weeks."* – **Doug from Salt Lake City, Utah**

And…

*"Your presentation showed me the **simple solution** to my diabetes, and you had **the science to back it up**.*

I thought I'd be stuck with Type 2 diabetes forever. But now I've been diabetes-free almost 18 months.

My doctor was shocked when I told him that I hadn't needed an insulin shot for weeks. He had to test my blood sugar himself to believe it.

The best part is, I used what I discovered… to **jumpstart my pancreas** *and reverse my diabetes in just 17 days!"* **Andrew from Battleground, Washington**

…after reading this book, you can see how it truly is possible to reverse diabetes forever.

But you will have also realized that it can involve adjusting most of your daily habits and routines and that in itself can be a daunting prospect.

It's a complicated life change, and most of us people struggle with one or two small daily adjustments.

What if there was an easier way?

A short cut to destroying diabetes forever?

Well, now there is…

Visit the URL below to watch the video presentation:

pressroyale.com/shortcut

CONCLUSION

Consider this.

Diabetes is not a drug-fueled death sentence, despite what so-called Big Pharma would have you believe.

You can reverse diabetes.

You can live a longer, happier, and healthier life.

Diabetes has a negative effect on everybody it touches.

You can change that.

Show your loved ones and colleagues that you can beat it.

Prove it to yourself.

The greatest legacy anyone can have is to make a positive change to their world.

You can make this change.

Help yourself.

By making this change to your health, you will inspire others to do the same to their health.

Save your life.

Save their lives.

<u>You can do it.</u>

To your success,

Randall Vincent-Martin

P.S. Now you've reached the end of my first book, I would like to ask a little something of you.

Reader reviews are the lifeblood of any author's career.

For a humble typewriter-jockey like myself, getting reviews (especially on Amazon) means I can submit my books for advertising.

Which means I can actually sell a few copies from time to time - which is always a nice bonus :)

So every review really does means a lot to me.

Leaving a review is super easy:

1. Go to **pressroyale.com/rdreview**
2. Sign in to Amazon if prompted
3. Select a star rating
4. Write a few short words (or long words, I won't judge)
5. Click the 'submit' button

…and you'll make an old man very happy!

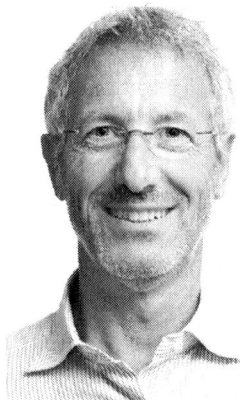

And you'll inspire me to continue writing books that help everyone through the daily struggles of diabetes.

Thanks again,

Randall

SHOPPING LIST

Essential Equipment

Blood Pressure Monitor pressroyale.com/pressure

Blood Glucose Monitor pressroyale.com/glucose

Cholesterol Analyzer pressroyale.com/cholesterol

Nicotine-Free Harmless Cigarette pressroyale.com/smoke

Healthy Foods

Agave pressroyale.com/agave

Stevia pressroyale.com/stevia

Organic Honey pressroyale.com/honey

Organic Vegetable Box pressroyale.com/veg

Books & DVDs

Diabetic Desserts Book pressroyale.com/dessert

Diabetic Exercise DVD pressroyale.com/dvd

LINKS

BMI Calculator

pressroyale.com/bmi

Diabetes Superfoods

pressroyale.com/superfoods

Diabetic Desserts

pressroyale.com/diabeticdesserts

Transformational Breath

pressroyale.com/breath

SUPPORT GROUPS

Diabetes Support

USA: pressroyale.com/dbsupportus

UK: pressroyale.com/dbsupportuk

Weight Loss Support

USA: pressroyale.com/wlsupportus

UK: pressroyale.com/wlsupportuk

Walking Groups

USA: pressroyale.com/walkus

UK: pressroyale.com/walkuk

Stop Smoking Support

USA: pressroyale.com/smokeus

UK: pressroyale.com/smokeuk

REFERENCES

Chapter 3: Axe, Dr. J. (2014, March 20). *10 Turmeric benefits superior to medications at reversing disease.* Retrieved July 28, 2016, from https://draxe.com/turmeric-benefits/

Chapter 6: Spiegel, A. (2008, January 3). *Hotel maids challenge the placebo effect.* Retrieved July 28, 2016, from npr.org/templates/story/story.php?storyId=17792517

Chapter 6: Werner, R. (2008). *A massage therapist's guide to pathology (LWW massage therapy & Bodywork educational series)* (4th ed.) (568 – 570). Baltimore, MD: Wolters Kluwer/Lippincott Williams & Wilkins.

Chapter 8: Avena, N (2010). *A sweet problem: Princeton researchers find that high-fructose corn syrup prompts considerably more weight gain.* Retrieved August 1, 2016, from princeton.edu/main/news/archive/S26/91/22K07/

FREE KINDLE BOOKS

Love free stuff?

Love Kindle books?

Join The Press Royale Kindle Book Club!

You'll get a weekly email with download links for quality titles on every topic imaginable.

It's 100% free, and super simple to join.

Just visit our site below and enter your email address.

pressroyale.com

You'll NEVER be short of something to read – ever again!

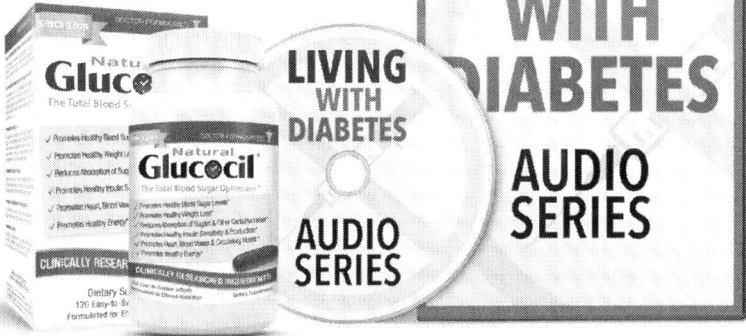

Every copy of this book comes packed with these valuable bonuses:

BONUS #1
Glucocil Natural Blood Sugar Optimizer - **15 DAY SAMPLE**

BONUS #2
"Living With Diabetes" Audio Series - **FREE INSTANT DOWNLOAD**

BONUS #3
"Diabetes & You" Weekly Newsletter - **FREE INSTANT ACCESS**

Simply visit the special URL below and enter your name & email address for instant access.

pressroyale.com/claim

ISBN: 1536890855
ISBN-13: 978-1536890853

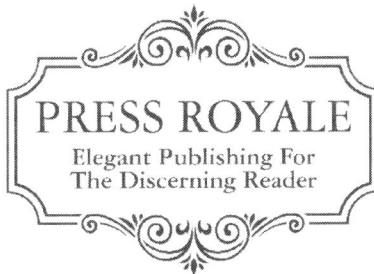

Printed in Great Britain
by Amazon